Information Circular 9499

Guidelines for the Development of a New Miner Training Curriculum

By Charles Vaught, Ph.D., and Launa G. Mallett, Ph.D.

DEPARTMENT OF HEALTH AND HUMAN SERVICES
Centers for Disease Control and Prevention
National Institute for Occupational Safety and Health
Pittsburgh Research Laboratory
Pittsburgh, PA

January 2008

Disclaimer

Mention of any company or product does not constitute endorsement by the National Institute for Occupational Safety and Health (NIOSH). In addition, citations to Web sites external to NIOSH do not constitute NIOSH endorsement of the sponsoring organizations or their programs or products. Furthermore, NIOSH is not responsible for the content of these Web sites.

Ordering Information

To receive documents or other information about occupational safety and health topics, contact NIOSH at

> Telephone: **1–800–CDC–INFO** (1–800–232–4636)
> TTY: 1–888–232–6348
> e-mail: cdcinfo@cdc.gov
>
> or visit the NIOSH Web site at **www.cdc.gov/niosh**.

For a monthly update on news at NIOSH, subscribe to NIOSH *eNews* by visiting **www.cdc.gov/niosh/eNews**.

DHHS (NIOSH) Publication No. 2008–105

January 2008

SAFER • HEALTHIER • PEOPLE™

CONTENTS

Page

GUIDELINES FOR THE DEVELOPMENT
OF A NEW MINER TRAINING CURRICULUM

By Charles Vaught, Ph.D.,[1] and Launa G. Mallett, Ph.D.[2]

ABSTRACT

This report is intended to help mine safety trainers better prepare to teach the influx of new underground coal miners who are entering the industry. This is done by identifying two different approaches to instruction and discussing the ways they may affect how well prepared new hires are to deal with a dynamic and hazardous workplace. One approach is based on the use of a syllabus. Those using a syllabus are more likely to rely on lecturing or direct instruction. This is a good way to get across factual information, but does not provide a context within which miners can fit the discrete facts so that they form an integrated whole set of concepts, principles, and skills. The other approach is based on the use of a curriculum. Those using a curriculum may be more likely to help miners integrate concepts and skills that give them an overall picture of the complex mining environment and how they fit into the workplace. This will better prepare them for the decision-making and problem-solving activities that will help them work safely and productively.

---

[1]Senior research scientist.
[2]Lead research scientist.
Pittsburgh Research Laboratory, National Institute for Occupational Safety and Health, Pittsburgh, PA.

INTRODUCTION

With the coal boom of the late 1960s and early 1970s, there was an increased demand for mining personnel. This resulted in a large influx of inexperienced individuals into the nation's mines. There, they became part of a system in which more experienced miners had traditionally mentored new hires, teaching them "mine wiseness" and how to be safe, productive workers. Unfortunately, as more and more new people entered the workplace, there were relatively fewer experienced hands to do the mentoring. Add to this the fact that older workers were retiring, and the situation became critical.

Given the makeup of the workforce, therefore, training assumed a greater role in preparing new miners to do their jobs. This role was underscored by the Federal Mine Safety and Health Act of 1977 (Public Law 91–173, as amended by Public Law 95–164), which created 30 CFR[3] 48. Part 48 sets a minimum of 40 hours of new miner training, 32 of which can take place in the classroom. Provision was also made for 8 hours of annual refresher training, which sets forth a dozen courses of study.

These courses present basic factual information about such things as statutory rights, mine gases, electrical hazards, etc. Simply relating facts and figures, however, does not prepare the individual to work safely when he or she enters the mine. Again, it is best if there are experienced workers who can put factual information obtained in the classroom into the context of the workplace. By the early 1980s, with the downturn in hiring, there were once again experienced miners to mentor the few individuals being hired, and the type of training received by these new hires was normally not an issue.

Today, mining has come full circle. The industry's demand for new employees is at a level not seen since the 1970s. In addition, "baby boomers" are retiring from the mines in ever-increasing numbers. Since the start of the new millennium, industry experts have been looking at how these factors may impact the industry and what should be done to prepare for the changes that have already started. There is one certainty: the large numbers of miners currently being hired and anticipated in the coming years will not have the luxury of a slow introduction to the workplace under the supervision of experienced mentors. Instead, crews made up largely of relatively inexperienced workers will have to rely on their training. It is in their classes that new employees should be taught what it means to be miners. Here they ought to encounter, perhaps for the first time, concepts of occupational safety and health and practical methods for protecting themselves. One area that needs to be explored, therefore, is how new miners have been trained in the past and how they might come to be trained in the future.

This report presents a model curriculum for Part 48 new miner training. Basic elements of the model are abstracted from the best practices of industry trainers, augmented by findings from research by the National Institute for Occupational Safety and Health's (NIOSH) Pittsburgh Research Laboratory. Taken as a whole, the model can serve as a guideline for applied curriculum development. Trainers will be able to tailor the components to their own needs.

SYLLABUS VERSUS CURRICULUM

Part 48 is a double-edged sword. On one hand, it mandates a core of courses containing content about which miners should be knowledgeable. On the other hand, the courses are presented in such a way that they form an incantation that may be interpreted by trainers as a listing of all the factual information they need to impart to trainees (usually as discrete bits of

---

[3] *Code of Federal Regulations.* See CFR in references.

knowledge) in order to comply with the law. The use of Part 48 courses to derive a list of factual topics for instruction produces a syllabus. Syllabus is defined as "an outline or a summary of the main points of a text, lecture, or course of study" (Microsoft Bookshelf 2000). "A syllabus lists subjects to be taught and the topics within each subject, without indicating the objectives or how it will be implemented" [Temu and Kasolo 2001]. New miner training programs that are based on syllabi focus mainly on content to the exclusion of broader overarching concepts. The problem with teaching this way is that it is context-free. There is no "big picture" within which to fit the bits of information so that they form a whole. This is necessary in order to build concepts and cognitive skills that better prepare the new miner for the decision-making and problem-solving strategies that are essential to work safely and productively in the complex mining environment.

An alternative approach to new miner training is to develop a curriculum based on Part 48, but which goes beyond mere compliance with the law. One way in which curriculum may be defined is: "a plan of instruction that details what students are to know, how they are to learn it, what the teacher's role is, and the context in which learning and teaching will take place" [Learning Point Associates 2002]. Although there is no particular accepted definition of curriculum, this one evokes many of the elements:

(1) Planning – Curriculum encompasses all the learning that is planned and guided by the trainer [Rogers and Taylor 1998];
(2) Objectives – The key to curriculum, objectives stipulate what the trainee is to come away with in terms of new knowledge and skills;
(3) Delivery – How trainees learn may range from lecture, to hands-on practice, to media-based training;
(4) Content – What is to be delivered;
(5) Teacher's role – The trainer may assume an active and directive role, act as a facilitator, or simply serve as an expert partner to the trainees; and
(6) Context – Some notions of curriculum picture training as a social endeavor that may be carried on in many settings, as long as it is planned and directed [Smith 2000].

One important element that is missing in the above definition of curriculum is evaluation. Curriculum development should include a plan for evaluating the curriculum as a whole, including feedback from learners. As can be seen, there are many more things that make up a curriculum than a simple list of topics to be taught. Curriculum suggests that learning is a long-term process that takes place both inside and outside the classroom. In terms of new miner training, it provides a way to integrate what is learned in the classroom with the day-to-day activities that occur in the workplace.

The remainder of this report is organized in the following way: (1) a short discussion of new miner training using a syllabus approach, (2) examination of a comprehensive syllabus used by the Midwestern Department of Mine Safety and Training,[4] (3) consideration of the likely role of the trainer when he or she is relying on a syllabus, (4) discussion of new miner training from the perspective of a curriculum, (5) an examination of a model curriculum used by a major coal company operating in western Pennsylvania, and (6) a discussion of the possible role of a trainer when using a curriculum. Because evaluation should be a part of curriculum development but often is not, there is a section discussing its importance. Finally, there is a summary and conclusions section that integrates the ideas put forth in the report.

---

[4]This is a pseudonym to ensure anonymity.

USING A SYLLABUS

Even in the university, people confuse syllabus with curriculum [Smith 2000]. Perhaps the best way to conceptualize their relationship is to start with the fact that they are not two totally different things. Rather, a syllabus can be part of a curriculum and shares some elements with the broader concept (such as planning, for instance). Where syllabus differs is in the narrowness of its scope. Essentially, a syllabus is merely a comprehensive listing of the content of a body of work that is to be imparted to trainees in the form of writing or lecture (or both). The listing of Part 48 courses compiled by the Midwestern Department of Mine Safety and Training (see Appendix A) is an excellent example of a syllabus, although it is simply a repeat of the mandatory courses laid out in Part 48. Since the syllabus is taken in its entirety from the list in Part 48, it is unclear how much actual planning went into its compilation. It is also unclear how the content is to be conveyed to the trainees or what role the instructor will play in the process. Finally, there is no provision for evaluation to take place.

The Department did, however, author a separate document that articulates a goal and objective for the Department's Part 48 training. The overall goal is to reduce injuries and fatalities by educating new miners in the safety and health aspects of the environment they soon will enter. The Department's objective is to train the miners in the required subjects listed in Part 48, including any additional topics that the Mine Safety and Health Administration's (MSHA) District Manager deems necessary.

Given the Department's goal, its stated objective misses the mark. The ABC's of objectives are: (1) identify the audience, (2) draft a statement of the behavior that is expected from the trainee once he or she has been trained, and (3) specify the conditions under which the trainee will demonstrate his or her knowledge or skills [Clark 2000]. Objectives are the end of the training process—that which a trainee must achieve given what the trainer states is to be learned [Texas Tech 2007]. The Department's objective, rather than spelling out what the trainee is to do in order to contribute to the reduction of injuries and fatalities, instead relates what the trainers will do in their role of instructors. In other words, their stated objective is actually the means to an end rather than the end itself.

Given that the Department's intent is to reduce injuries and fatalities, an objective, rather than focusing on compliance, should be a precise statement of what behavior the new hire would engage in as part of his or her role as a miner [Clark 2000]. For instance, an objective might be: a new miner (audience) will identify and avoid (behaviors) unstable roof given his or her involvement in the workplace (condition). Note that the behaviors are given as action verbs because they need to be observable and, in some instances, measurable. That is the only way the trainer can tell if the objective has been met.

One activity the Department engages in to enhance the syllabus and account, at least partially, for the mining context is to tailor its presentations to address the characteristics of the mine where the new workers will be employed. The Department's instructors do this by first visiting the mine site and performing an audit of conditions. Then, before their program is implemented, they discuss any particular training needs with mine management and the operation's safety representative. This allows the trainer to understand the workings of the mine and any problems that might be encountered. Thus, the trainer will be able to make his or her class mine-specific.

The instructional model that best reflects the role a trainer is most likely to take if he or she uses a syllabus is the one most prevalent in industry [Caudron 2000] and is how miners have traditionally been taught. It is characterized by direct instruction, in which a trainer assumes an active and directive role. He or she maintains control of the pace, sequencing, and content of the lesson [Baumann 1998], acting as a conduit for factual information that the student is responsible for grasping. Palincsar [1998] noted that while research supports the notion that this is an effective way to teach factual content, there is little evidence that this type of instruction transfers to higher-order cognitive skills such as reasoning and problem-solving. Nor, according to Peterson and Wallberg [1979], is there much evidence that it results in the flexibility individuals need in order to use effective strategies in uncertain contexts. Mining is hazardous in part because the worker's physical environment is dynamic, or constantly changing. The need to continually respond to such a dynamic work environment places individuals at risk. The constantly changing conditions require a skilled and vigilant workforce that can quickly adapt to the new hazards and changing risks [Scharf et al. 2001]. This has implications for how workers can best be trained. In essence, direct instruction as an instructional model is not the best way to train workers in higher-order concepts and skills because it "has limitations related to the influences of human thinking and social interaction as these apply to both individual and group behavior. The model is also less adequate for explaining [and changing] behavior in the more open, self-directed situations that describe [dynamic work settings]" [Cole 2002].

USING A CURRICULUM

Part 48 mandates a list of courses that are to be taught to new miners. As such, it is a syllabus. Therefore, a trainer wishing to construct a curriculum for new miner training begins with topics already assigned. The question then becomes, "Why try to develop a curriculum; why not just use the syllabus that is provided (as did the Midwestern Department of Mine Safety and Training)?" The short answer is that, although the curriculum will be content-driven, it does not negate the need to devise a teaching method that will get the information across in such a way that the trainees become active learners of not just the rules contained in Part 48, but their meaning and how to apply them to cope with the exigencies of the mine's dynamic work setting. Besides, content is malleable. It means different things to different people depending on their life experiences, how the instructor chooses to deliver the content, what is in the message, how it is received and interpreted, and whether it contains information they can take back to the workplace.

In addition to content and teaching method are those other elements that make up a curriculum, including planning, objectives, delivery method, content, teacher's role, context, and evaluation. A carefully designed and well thought-out curriculum may include all these factors [Unwin 1997]. However, there is a core that is most important: (1) objectives, because if trainers do not know where they are going, they will not know if and when they get there; (2) appropriate delivery method, because it is the vehicle that carries the content; (3) appropriate content, because it is necessary in order to achieve objectives; and (4) evaluation, because it tells whether the process is working and objectives have been met.

> "If we could first know where we are, and whither we are tending, we could then better judge what to do, and how to do it." —Abraham Lincoln

The overall purpose of a new miner training curriculum is to help trainers provide young/inexperienced miners a grounding in the context of those core courses that are mandated under 30 CFR 48.5 (see Appendix A). It is the notion that trainees should be grounded in the mining context that guides a well thought-out curriculum. 30 CFR 48.5(a) states that new miner training "shall be conducted in conditions which as closely as practicable duplicate actual underground conditions." Obviously, a classroom does not do a very good job of duplicating an underground coal mine. Some activities that take place in the classroom, however, can evoke activities that occur in the workplace. The trainee may be given the opportunity to work with others to solve problems taken from actual workplace predicaments, for instance. In doing so, he or she can learn such things as some of the occupational jargon, the rules that apply in certain situations, and perhaps gain an understanding of the tools that miners use.

The rationale for such a curriculum is that it provides a way to involve trainees more in the learning process. Unlike a curriculum built around direct instruction in which the trainer controls the pace, sequencing, and content of the lesson, this curriculum is based upon the notion that trainees should be more proactive in solving problems taken from workplace situations. The focus is less on the trainer and more on the trainees who generally are given the opportunity to work together in their problem-solving activities. This is important because they must work together in the workplace.

> "Tell me, and I will forget. Show me, and I may remember. Involve me, and I will understand." —Confucius

A company that operates mines in western Pennsylvania has put together an exemplary 80-hour new miner training program. Over the 10-day course, the trainees divide their time between the classroom and an underground training section.

On the first day, as part of their orientation, the trainees are prepared to go underground. The objective of the preparation is to ensure that each trainee has an understanding of how the classroom instruction is combined with hands-on underground training. During the second half of day 1 and the first half of day 2, the trainees are instructed in their roles as miners, how to read a map and evacuate in an emergency, the use of self-rescue and respiratory devices, cleanup and rock dusting requirements, securing the workplace, and other topics to prepare them to go underground. After lunch on day 2, they are equipped for work inside. As part of the session on entering and leaving the mine, transportation, and communication, the trainees must demonstrate the ability to use the mine's hand scanner to check in and check out and are trained in the operation of the elevator, phones, and pagers. They are then given a walking tour of the mine, which takes them to the training section for a preview of the work to be performed during the in-mine training sessions. Finally, they travel to the elevator where they are required to explain how to cage to the surface.

The morning of the third day begins with health and safety aspects of assigned tasks. The students are expected to know the hazards of each assigned task and procedures to minimize them. During a session on transportation and communication, the students learn methods of safely transporting people and materials into and out of the mine, traffic controls, types of communication, and warning and directional signs in use. Next, they have a session on roof control and ventilation in which they are required to demonstrate an understanding of how to remove or support loose roof and ribs, as well as the procedures for maintaining and controlling ventilation. Lastly, the trainees are required to be able to identify the mine's ventilation systems and devices, how air gets to the face, mine and section ventilation, and methane and other gases and how they are controlled.

In the afternoon of the third day, the trainees enter the mine and travel to the training section. Once there, they are introduced to the work environment—basic job skills and work hardening (what they will need to do physically). They are made aware of various methods used to address mine hazards. For instance, each employee will demonstrate the sight, sound, and vibration method for checking the roof. The trainee will also demonstrate proper scaling procedures, shovel along the ribs, and rock dust the area. On the way out to the elevator, there will be a discussion of manholes, switches, and guidelines for walking along the haulage.

As stated previously, the core of a curriculum is made up of a system of objectives, delivery method, content, and evaluation. There are some other elements that complement the core in order to round out a curriculum, which were also listed earlier. As Appendix B shows, the instructors at this company have developed a lesson plan (planning) that has many of the various elements that define a curriculum. The objectives detail the learning outcomes expected from participation in the curriculum. Teaching methods (delivery) are spelled out in the lesson plan. Subject matter designates the content the curriculum deals with. The trainer's role as lecturer, demonstrator, discussion leader, and evaluator is suggested in the lesson plan. Context is ensured by the classroom/underground experience. Finally, the lesson plan indicates how evaluation will be carried out, although the plan itself stops at individual assessment. Assessment bears the same relation to evaluation as syllabus does to curriculum. Hanson et al. [1996] note that "the purpose of student assessment, either through observable performance, product development, or traditional paper and pencil tests, is to provide data to the instructor [and the learner] indicating to what degree the performance objectives have been mastered." As part of their overall program, however, the instructors also conduct some basic evaluation in the form of feedback from trainees (see Appendix D). "Evaluation is the process of determining whether programs—or certain aspects of programs—are appropriate, adequate, effective, and efficient and, if not, how to make them so" [Deniston and Rosenstock 1970]. Evaluation will be discussed in more detail later. In sum, though, for all practical purposes, Appendix B identifies a curriculum.

Appendix C contains the tasks and duties for the training section. It does for the work underground what Appendix B does for classroom training, except it is not set up like a curriculum instructional plan. Rather, it is a listing of topics covering the expected behaviors that accompany each assigned task.

The approach to learning and instruction that may be taken by a trainer using a curriculum recognizes that knowledge and skills reside not just in the heads of individuals, but in shared group practice [Lave 1988]. Learning these knowledge and skill sets requires an ongoing interaction with the work at hand and with those doing the work. With assisted practice, a person learns the strategies for completing a task, which then becomes part of his or her problem-solving inventory—knowledge that may be applied to new situations [Wilhelm et al. 2001]. "Under this view, safety education becomes a process of helping…workers to better understand the constraints and plights under which they work and to better identify and use the resources, knowledge, and tools available to their social group. The goal is to help the group become more proactive in improving health and safety within their community of workers" [Cole 2002].

The training approach, rather than being teacher-centered, as in direct instruction, is learning-centered. Also, rather than putting the responsibility for learning on the student alone, learning-centered instruction is two-sided and requires mutual effort and responsibility on the part of both learners and teachers. The classroom (or work setting) becomes a "community of practice" in which the teacher is a more expert partner providing leadership and assistance to those who are less skilled [Wilhelm et al. 2001]. These communities of practice are oriented toward solving problems in a real context. Because of its problem-solving orientation, the notion of a community of practice composed of learners and more expert partners fits well the needs of teaching and learning in a dynamic work setting.

The purpose of a problem-solving approach is, in part, to explore ways in which the training classroom can be made to more nearly reflect the workplace context. This is because in the traditional classroom, with its direct instruction, there is a disconnect between training and what Brown et al. [1989] termed "authentic activity." Authentic activity is, essentially, the ordinary practice that takes place within a workplace culture. It is the culture, made up of everything from occupational jargon, to formal and informal rules, to the tools practitioners use, that imparts meaning and purpose to the people who share it: "Authentic activity, as we have argued, is important for learners, because it is the only way they gain access to the standpoint that enables practitioners to act meaningfully and purposefully" [Brown et al. 1989]. Too often, training activity is very different from authentic activity because it is very different from what authentic practitioners do. The problem then becomes one of how to bring authenticity into the classroom.

Brown et al. [1989] used the notion of "cognitive apprenticeship" to show how this might be accomplished. In essence, a cognitive apprentice learns by working with others to solve problems taken from activities that occur in the community of practice. There are two implications of this approach. First, the learning that takes place is collaborative in nature. This is important because people must work together on the job. Thus, they must be given the situated opportunity to develop those skills. Second, the problems are "real" in their use of authentic activity and so must be presented in realistic fashion. Prior NIOSH and University of Kentucky research has suggested some ways this can be done. For instance, researchers have developed and field-tested simulations that were constructed by first listening to and learning from an experienced workforce, then combining this practical knowledge with empirical injury surveillance data and safety research findings [Cole et al. 1988]. Researchers from the NIOSH Spokane Research Laboratory have incorporated authentic storytelling into safety training [Cullen and Fein 2005]. Both of these approaches function to involve the learner in the situation and help prepare him or her for on-the-job contingencies.

EVALUATION

As mentioned earlier, curriculum development should also include a plan for evaluating the curriculum as a whole, including feedback from learners. Although individual assessment can be seen as part of evaluation, much more is involved. This section focuses on three other aspects of evaluation: feedback from learners, changes in behavior, and effects on the organization.

Trainee reactions are the easiest kind of data to gather. That it not to say they are not important. If trainees do not see value in the training, they are not likely to translate course objectives into useful knowledge and skills. When trainees find a course uninteresting, they will be less motivated to learn the material being covered. While positive trainee reactions do not ensure that objectives are met, negative reactions guarantee a less-than-fully-successful transfer of knowledge and skills. The following is an excerpt from a questionnaire that accompanies a paper-and-pencil simulation:

	Strongly Agree	Agree	Disagree	Strongly Disagree
This scenario could happen in real life	1	2	3	4
I learned something new from this exercise	1	2	3	4

Measuring a change in behavior must be done outside the classroom and with sufficient time elapsed for knowledge and skills to have been tried out in the workplace. The most elaborate plan for evaluating behavior would include an untrained subgroup and a trained subgroup with detailed testing in their workplaces before and after training. This type of evaluation is resource-intensive and would not be practical for all training sessions. But less intensive strategies can yield valuable results:

> Something beats nothing, and I encourage trainers to at least do some evaluation of behavior, even if it isn't elaborate or scientific. Simply ask a few people: "Are you doing anything different on the job because you attended the training program?" If the answer is yes, ask, "Can you briefly describe what you are doing and how it is working out? If you are not doing anything different, can you tell me why? Did you learn anything that you can use on the job?" [Kirkpatrick 2001]

Another strategy is to talk with the trainee's supervisor about any behavioral changes they have observed since the training was completed. As can be seen, this type of evaluation can be difficult because it may be conducted months after the training has been completed. Thus, it is important to devise an evaluation plan when the course is being planned. Time must be scheduled for the followup data collection so it will not interfere with future training activities and projects.

The most difficult evaluation to perform is determining how training affects the organization. This strategy should be undertaken when the value of the training or the training program to the overall organization needs to be assessed. To conduct such an evaluation, it is important to clearly define the tangible results to be measured, such as a decrease in workplace hazards, an increase in the use of personal protective equipment, a reduction in maintenance costs, or an increase in production per shift. Once the desired result is identified, a means to measure changes is needed. Next, factors other than training that could influence the change should be identified so that they can be ruled out as the source of change, if possible. Finally, evidence that the training did cause the change being studied should be identified—and it is usually necessary to be satisfied with evidence rather than proof, because proof is hard to find [Kirkpatrick 2001].

In sum, the only way to determine whether or not training is of value is to evaluate it. When objectives for the training are clearly defined, an evaluation plan can be designed to measure the training's effectiveness at achieving those goals. Sometimes company managers or outside organizations require evaluation data to assess a training program. Even when such outside influences are not present, it is in the best interests of a trainer to gather evaluation data routinely to assess course content, delivery methods, and teaching skills. If a course is to be repeated, evaluation can guide changes to improve future sessions. If the course will not be repeated, evaluation could focus on the skills of the instructor, with the results used for professional development of that trainer. The important thing is to decide what can and should be learned during training evaluations and then design a strategy to meet that goal.

SUMMARY AND CONCLUSIONS

These guidelines began with the fact that new miners entering the workforce today will enter an environment that is dynamic and hazardous. Because there will be a scarcity of experienced miners to mentor these new hires, the training they get assumes great importance. It is in training sessions that they need to acquire those concepts and cognitive skills that will help them make decisions and develop problem-solving strategies in order to become safe and productive workers.

The authors next discussed two general approaches to training. An approach based on the use of a syllabus might serve well to transmit basic information in discrete bits. However, an approach based on curriculum is better suited to help trainees place the information into a meaningful context. This is important because workers need to understand their work and job performance in the overall scheme of things in order to better deal with their environment.

The guidelines point out that each approach has a preferred teaching method associated with it. If the goal is compliance, a directed teaching method is the best fit with a syllabus. If the goal is for miners to become grounded in the mining context, an effective teaching method is one that helps workers better understand how to solve problems using the tools and resources at hand in their work environment [Cole 2002].

A curriculum is a better approach for preparing new miners to work underground because it has components lacking in a syllabus. Chief among these is a set of objectives. An objective, properly stated, identifies a performance outcome—what the learner is to do, not what facts the learner learns [Clark 2000]. Objectives should be in line with stated goals. If the goal is to reduce injuries and fatalities, a proper objective would identify a specific set of behaviors that can contribute to this reduction. As discussed earlier, an objective should be precise enough that people will understand what it is and be able to recognize when it is met [Clark 2000]. Objectives are so important that it can be argued the other elements of a curriculum do not matter when there is no objective. Simply put, "If you don't know where you are going, how do you know when you've arrived?" [Landau 2001].

Evaluation was treated as a special case because it is so often ignored in the process of developing a curriculum. Evaluation is critical, however, because it is what determines if the training program is "appropriate, adequate, effective and efficient and, if not, how to make [it] so" [Deniston and Rosenstock 1970].

In sum, these guidelines have made a simple argument: the trainer should (1) be fully conversant with the content domain (syllabus) that is required, (2) develop appropriate and observable objectives, (3) adopt a teaching method that will help trainees problem-solve in order to meet these objectives, and (4) evaluate the process. The outcome will be new miners who are better equipped cognitively and skill-wise to deal with the exigencies of their workplace.

REFERENCES

Baumann J [1998]. Direct instruction reconsidered. J Reading Behav *31*:712–718.

Brown J, Collins A, Duguid P [1989]. Situated cognition and the culture of learning. Educ Res *18*(1):32–42.

Caudron S [2000]. Learners speak out. Train Dev *54*(4):52–57.

CFR. Code of federal regulations. Washington DC: U.S. Government Printing Office, Office of the Federal Register.

Clark D [2000]. More on learning objectives. [http://www.nwlink.com/~donclark/hrd/objectives.htm]. Date accessed: October 2007.

Cole HP [2002]. Cognitive-behavioral approaches to farm community safety education: a conceptual analysis. J Agric Saf Health *8*(2):145–159.

Cole HP, Mallett LG, Haley JV, Berger PK, Lacefield WE, Wasielewski RD, Lineberry GT, Wala AM [1988]. Research and evaluation methods for measuring nonroutine mine health and safety skills. Vol. I. Lexington, KY: University of Kentucky. U.S. Bureau of Mines contract No. H0348040). NTIS No. PB 89–196646/AS.

Cullen ET, Fein AH [2005]. Tell me a story: why stories are essential to effective safety training. Spokane, WA: U.S. Department of Health and Human Services, Public Health Service, Centers for Disease Control and Prevention, National Institute for Occupational Safety and Health, DHHS (NIOSH) Publication No. 2005–152, RI 9664.

Deniston O, Rosenstock I [1970]. Evaluating health programs. Public Health Rep *85*(9):835–840.

Hanson D, Maushak N, Schlosser C, Anderson M, Sorenson C, Simonson M [1996]. Distance education: review of the literature. 2nd ed. Ames, IA: Iowa State University, Research Institute for Studies in Education.

Kirkpatrick D [2001]. The four-level evaluation process. In: Ukens L, ed. What smart trainers know: the secrets of success from the world's foremost experts. San Francisco, CA: Jossey-Bass/Pfeiffer, pp. 122–132.

Landau V [2001]. Developing an effective online course: developing goals and objectives. [http://roundworldmedia.com/cvc/module4/topic4.html]. Date accessed: October 2007.

Lave J [1988]. Cognition in practice: mind, mathematics, and culture in everyday life. Cambridge, U.K.: Cambridge University Press.

Learning Point Associates [2002]. Glossary of education terms and acronyms. [http://www.ncrel.org/sdrs/areas/misc/glossary.htm]. Date accessed: October 2007.

Palincsar A [1998]. Social constructivist perspectives on teaching. Annu Rev Psychol *49*:345–380.

Peterson PL, Wallberg HJ, eds. [1979]. Research on teaching. Berkeley, CA: McCutchan.

Rogers A, Taylor P [1998]. Participatory curriculum development in agricultural education: a training guide. Rome, Italy: Food and Agricultural Organization of the United Nations (FAO).

Scharf T, Vaught C, Kidd P, Steiner LJ, Kowalski KM, Wiehagen WJ, Rethi LL, Cole HP [2001]. Toward a typology of dynamic and hazardous work environments. Hum Ecol Risk Assess *7*(7):1827–1841.

Smith MK [2000]. Curriculum theory and practice. In: The encyclopaedia of informal education. [http://www.infed.org/biblio/b-curric.htm]. Date accessed: October 2007.

Temu AB, Kasolo W [2001]. Reviewing curricula – rationale, process and outputs: ANAFE experience with the DACUM method in Africa. In: Expert Consultation on Forestry Education (Rabat, Morocco, October 17–19, 2001). Rome, Italy: Food and Agricultural Organization of the United Nations (FAO).

Texas Tech [2007]. Developing teaching objectives. Lubbock, TX: Texas Tech University, Department of Agricultural Education and Communications. [http://www.depts.ttu.edu/aged/aged2300/DevelopingObjectives.pdf]. Date accessed: October 2007.

Unwin DJ [1997]. NCGIA core curriculum in geographic information science. Curriculum design for GIS. [http://www.ncgia.ucsb.edu/giscc/units/u159/u159.html]. Date accessed: October 2007.

Wilhelm JD, Baker TN, Dube J [2001]. Strategic reading: guiding students to lifelong literacy, 6–12. Portsmouth, NH: Heinemann.

APPENDIX A.—A SYLLABUS FOR MINER TRAINING

Surface

A. Statutory Rights of Miners and Their Representative under the Act
   1. Statutory rights of miners and their representative under the Act
   2. Discussion of Section 2 of the Act
   3. The line of authority of supervision
   4. The miners' representative
   5. Responsibilities of the supervisor and miners' representative
   6. Introduction to company rules
   7. Procedures for reporting hazards
B. Self-Rescue and Respiratory Devices
   1. Instruction in the use, care, and maintenance of the type of devices used at the mine
   2. Demonstration of the complete donning procedure
   3. Fit testing and the hazards if it is not done properly
   4. Discussion of the hazards of and prevention of silicosis
C. Transportation Controls and Communication Systems
   1. Riding conveyances
   2. Transportation of miners, materials, and explosives
   3. Use of mine communication systems
   4. Warning signals, signs, and directional signs used at the mine
   5. Powered haulage safety tips
D. Introduction to the Work Environment
   1. Discussion of the processes and type of mining used at the mine
   2. The company will be required to provide the majority of this subject.
E. Escape and Emergency Evacuation Plans; Fire Warning and Firefighting
   1. Review of the escape procedures and routes
   2. Review of the firefighting and emergency evacuation plans
   3. Instruction in the fire warning systems
F. Ground Control; Working in Areas of Highwalls, Water Hazards, Pits and Spoil Banks; Illumination and Night Work
   1. Highwalls and Ground Control Plans will be discussed.
   2. Procedures for working safely around highwalls
   3. Procedures for working around water
   4. Procedures for working around spoil banks
   5. Nighttime hazards identified and procedures for working after dark
   6. Site preparation and safety around highwalls
G. Health
   1. Instruction in how and why dust, noise, and other health measurements are taken and what they mean to the miner
   2. Discussion on the possible health hazards at the mine

3. Health controls in place at the mine are discussed.
    a. Silicosis
    b. Noise
    c. Winter weather alert
    d. Heat stress
    e. Hygiene
4. Health provisions of the Act are explained.
5. Warning labels and Material Safety Data Sheets (MSDSs) explained

H. Hazard Recognition
1. Normal mining hazards will be discussed.
2. Explosives, their use and hazards discussed
3. The operator will provide the majority of this class.

I. Electrical Hazards
1. Recognition and avoidance of electrical hazards
2. High-voltage dangers
3. Power center dangers
4. Grounding
5. Ground fault interruption
6. Substations
7. Disconnects
8. Lockout/tagout

J. First Aid
1. Primary survey
2. Secondary survey
3. CPR
4. Bandaging and splinting
5. Transportation

K. Explosives
1. Review and instruction in the use and danger of explosives
2. Hazards in the handling and transportation of explosives
3. Day boxes and magazines

L. Health and Safety Aspects of the Tasks Assigned
    This class will be provided by the operator.

M. Such other courses as may be required by the MSHA District Manager based on the circumstances and conditions found at the mine
1. Powered haulage safety
2. Fall prevention
3. Personal protective devices
4. Health and hygiene
5. Confined space entry
6. Hazardous materials handling
7. Materials handling

Underground

A. Statutory Rights of Miners and Their Representative Under the Act
   1. Statutory rights of miners and their representative under the Act
   2. Discussion of Section 2 of the Act
   3. The line of authority of supervision
   4. The miners' representative
   5. Responsibilities of the supervisor and miners' representative
   6. Introduction to company rules
   7. Procedures for reporting hazards
B. Self-Rescue and Respiratory Devices
   1. Instruction in the use, care, and maintenance of the type of devices used at the mine
   2. Demonstration of the complete donning procedure
   3. Fit testing and the hazards if it is not done properly
   4. Discussion of the hazards of and prevention of silicosis
C. Entering and Leaving the Mine; Transportation; Communications
   1. Procedures for entering and leaving the mine
   2. Check-in and checkout system
   3. Riding conveyances
   4. Transportation of miners, materials, and explosives
   5. Use of mine communication systems
   6. Warning signals, signs, and directional signs used at the mine
D. Introduction to the Work Environment
   1. Discussion of the processes and type of mining used at the mine
   2. The company will be required to provide the majority of this subject.
E. Mine Map; Escapeways; Emergency Evacuation; Barricading
   1. Review and discussion of the mine map
   2. Review of the escape procedures and routes
   3. Review of the firefighting and emergency evacuation plans
   4. Abandoned areas of the mine and their dangers
   5. Methods of barricading used at the mine
   6. Any refuge chambers and their locations
F. Roof, Ground Control, and Ventilation Plans
   1. Roof and Ground Control Plan will be discussed.
   2. Scaling techniques for the back, rib, and pillars
   3. Ventilation and its use in mining
   4. Discussion of the Mine Ventilation Plan
   5. Roof bolts and their use
   6. Examination of the working area
G. Health
   1. Instruction in how and why dust, noise, and other health measurements are taken and what the results mean to the miner
   2. Discussion on the possible health hazards at the mine

3. Health controls in place at the mine are discussed
    a. Silicosis
    b. Noise
    c. Winter weather alert
    d. Heat stress
    e. Hygiene
4. Health provisions of the Act are explained.
5. Warning labels and Material Safety Data Sheets (MSDSs) explained

H. Cleanup and Rock Dusting
   1. Housekeeping and the importance of cleanup at the mine
   2. The purpose of rock dusting
   3. Methods used at the mine
   4. The operator will provide portions of this class.

I. Hazard Recognition
   1. Normal mining hazards will be discussed.
   2. Explosives, their use and hazards discussed
   3. The operator will provide the majority of this class.

J. Electrical Hazards
   1. Recognition and avoidance of electrical hazards
   2. High-voltage dangers
   3. Power center dangers
   4. Grounding
   5. Ground fault interruption
   6. Substations
   7. Disconnects
   8. Lockout/tagout

K. First Aid
   1. Primary survey
   2. Secondary survey
   3. CPR
   4. Bandaging and splinting
   5. Transportation

L. Mine Gases
   1. Properties of gases
   2. Detection of and where to look for the various gases
   3. Hazards of gases: toxicity, explosive nature, and asphyxiation
   4. Avoidance and removal through ventilation

M. Health and Safety Aspects of the Tasks Assigned
   This class will be provided by the operator.

N. Such other courses as may be required by the MSHA District Manager based on the circumstances and conditions found at the mine
   1. Powered haulage safety
   2. Fall prevention
   3. Personal protective devices
   4. Health and hygiene
   5. Confined space entry
   6. Hazardous materials handling
   7. Materials handling

APPENDIX B.—NEW MINER TRAINING UNDERGROUND: 80 HOURS

	SUBJECT	OBJECTIVES	TEACHING METHODS	COURSE MATERIAL	EVALU-ATION METHODS
a.m.	Day 1 – a.m.				
1 HR Dept.	Welcome and overview of day 1, section 1	Introduction to HR, union, and management. Enrollment into all programs and benefits, coupled with a step-by-step introduction to benefits, policies, and procedures – 2 hours	Lecture and discussion.	Manuals and PowerPoint presentation, forms, and handouts.	Question, answer, and forms completed properly.
2 HR Dept.	Employee standards of conduct	Each miner will demonstrate his/her knowledge and understanding of the Employee Standards of Employment at the Pennsylvania operations.	PowerPoint and handout.	Handouts and PowerPoint slides.	Discussion with Q&A session.
3 HR and Mgt.	Organizational structure, union representation, chain of command	Introduce management and union officials and the organization structure —handling comments, complaints, and safety-related issues.	PowerPoint presentations, lecture, and discussions.	PowerPoint slides and handouts.	Open discussion with Q&A session.
4 HR Dept.	Hand scanner	Enroll each attendee in the hand-scan check-in and checkout process. The attendee will know how to scan in and out of the mine.	On-site training – Demon-stration and practice.	Hand scanner and log-on instructions.	Practice, demonstra-tion and actual log-in.
	Lunch				
p.m.	Day 1, Session 2	Preparation for underground (UG) on day 2			
1	Introduction to the training program – Course agenda and UG work	To ensure that each participant is aware of the nature of the program and his/her responsibilities as an employee, coupled with an overview and program agenda. Overview of the 10 days of training combining class-room with hands-on UG training.	Discussion and kickoff.	Handout of informational packets regarding the Pennsylvania operations and FCC.	Q&A session.
2	Your new role as a miner: history and tradition	To orient the new miners to the mine, its environment, and traditions. Show and discuss the first half of "The History of Mining" from The History Channel.	Video.	Video: "The History of Mining" (The History Channel).	Discussion.
3	Statutory rights Sec. 48.5(1) and an introduction to the authority and responsibility of supervisors and miners' reps – Sec. 48.6(3)	A comprehensive look at miners' rights and those of representatives of miners – aware of supervisor's responsibility and accountability under the Mine Act and company policy. Chain of command and union structure. Introduction to local officers was done in morning session with HR and management.	Videos, PowerPoint, discussion, demonstration.	Statutory Rights of Miners hand-out. Visual aids and handouts.	Oral response, discussion, quizzes.

	SUBJECT	OBJECTIVES	TEACHING METHODS	COURSE MATERIAL	EVALU-ATION METHODS
4	Mine map; escapeways; emergency evacuation; barricading – Sec. 48.5	Know how to read a mine map, when to evacuate a mine, which of the fire extinguishers to use in the event of a mine fire, and how to use the fire hose and nozzles. Cover guidelines as to when and when not to use them. **Mine-specific:** *Know where to report in the event of an emergency, how to get to safety from the workplace, the procedure in use to report a mine fire, how to erect barricades that isolate him/her from the rest of the mine, barricading rules, and how to signal rescuers. Oxygen requirements for barricading.*	Videos, PowerPoint, discussion, maps, program, and test.	Federal standards, audio-visual aids, mine map, company rules/policies. Federal guidelines for barricading and entrapment signals	Oral response, discussion, Q&A with quiz. Demonstration and handouts.
Day 2	Classroom				
1	Self-rescue and respiratory devices – Sec. 48.5(2)	Aware of the importance of using the proper type, correctly fitting respirator and the need for proper storage and maintenance. Understanding of when and how to apply a self-rescuer, what it protects against, the effect of high carbon monoxide on the user, and the danger of removing it. **Mine-specific:** *Will be trained in the proper use and care of the respiratory devices required at the mine, as well as self-rescuers.*	Videos, PowerPoint, discussion, and demonstration.	Federal standards, audio-visual aids, company rules	Oral response, discussion, quizzes, demonstration.
2	Cleanup; rock dusting – Sec. 48.5(8)	Finish on day 1 or carry over to day 2. Training in laws regarding rock dusting. Hazards of rock dusting around belts. Use of rock dust for firefighting. Mine cleanup plan and duties. This is preparation for going UG to begin general work in the training section. Rock dust requirements for intakes, returns, and belt lines.	Video, PowerPoint program on coal dust fires and explosions and rock dust in fire controls.	View video and discuss the process of rock dust, rock dusting, and purpose and application.	Q&A. Oral discussion and test.
3	Securing the workplace	Training on how to evaluate the work area for safety. What to look for and how to secure it. Roof and rib evaluation using sight, sound, and vibration method.	Video, PowerPoint discussion, and demonstration. Video clip of sounding roof and scaling roof and rib.	Trainees will be going underground for a walking tour to orient them in their assigned area and how to escape from that location.	Demonstration, Q&A session. Quiz.

	SUBJECT	OBJECTIVES	TEACHING METHODS	COURSE MATERIAL	EVALU-ATION METHODS
4	Proper lifting procedures	Mini-workshop on how to use proper lifting techniques in preparation to work on the training section.	PowerPoint presentation with pictures and demon-stration.	Each attendee will demon-strate the proper tech-niques for lifting and identify improper lifting tech-niques.	Demonstra-tion, quiz, Q&A.
	Lunch				
Day 2 UG 1	Equipping Miners	Assign lockers, outfit and have trainees dress for underground. Go over cap lights and how to maintain them. Review check-in and checkout, includ-ing hand scanners.	Demonstrate proper outfitting.	Observe each attendee as he/she dons cap, lamp, belt, leg bands, glasses, and gloves.	Demonstra-tion and Q&A.
UG	Entering and leaving the mine; transpor-tation and com-munication – Sec. 48.5(3)	*Demonstrate ability to use the mine's check-in and checkout system.* Enrolled in scanner system on day 1 session. Demonstrate the check-in and checkout system. Training in operation of elevator, phones, and pagers.	PowerPoint, discussion, mine tour.	Federal stand-ards, audio-visual aids, company rules/policies	Oral response, discussion, quizzes.
UG	Walking tour of the mine	Miners will tour area around bottom, travel to slope and main belt and haulage. Tour will take them to the training section for a preview of the work to be performed throughout the mine training sessions. *During work at training section, each trainee will receive the appropriate task training for the jobs performed.*	Tour, discus-sion, Q&A session.	Each attendee will explain the rules pertaining to each area traveled. Instructors will point out hazards, signals, rules, and policies regarding each area.	Demonstra-tion and discus-sions.
UG	Leaving the mine	Travel to elevator and explain caging to the surface			
Day 3	Classroom				
1	Health and safety aspects of assigned task – Sec. 48.5(13)	Aware of hazards associated with common underground mine tasks. **Mine-specific**: *Know the hazards of the assigned task and procedures to minimize them.*	Videos, PowerPoint discussion, demonstra-tion.	Federal stand-ards, audio-visual aids, company rules/policies, manufacturer information.	Oral response, demonstra-tion in mine.

	SUBJECT	OBJECTIVES	TEACHING METHODS	COURSE MATERIAL	EVALU-ATION METHODS
2	Transportation and communi-cation – Sec. 48.5(3)	Aware of applicable regulations regarding riding on or in mobile equipment. *Methods of transporting personnel and materials into and out of the mine, traffic controls, various types of communication, warning, and directional signs in use.*	Videos, PowerPoint, discussion, mine tour.	Federal stand-ards, audio-visual aids, company rules/policies.	Oral response, discussion, quiz.
3	Roof control and ventilation – Sec. 48.5(6)	Able to identify roof conditions and to demonstrate an understanding of methods of removing/supporting loose roof and ribs and procedures for maintaining and controlling ventilation. **Mine-specific:** *Demonstrate knowledge of roof/rib control procedures.*	Videos, PowerPoint, discussion, mine tour.	Federal stand-ards, audio-visual aids, Ground Con-trol Plan.	Oral response, discussion, quizzes.
4	Ventilation plans – Sec. 48.5(6)	Able to identify the various systems and devices, how air gets to the face, mine and section ventilation, methane, and other gases and how they are controlled. Introduction to the Ventilation Plan.	Video, PowerPoint, and handouts.	Federal and state stand-ards, Ventila-tion Plan, video, and PowerPoint presentation.	Quiz, maps completion exercise, oral response, and Q&A session
	Lunch				
UG	Enter mine	Check in and travel to section.			
UG	Introduction to work environ-ment – basic job skills and work hardening	Aware of methods used to address mine hazards. Each employee will demonstrate sight, sound, and vibration method. Demonstrate proper scaling procedures, shovel along ribs and rock dust the area.	Shovels, bars, pick, and rock dust.	Federal stand-ards, discus-sion, and demon-stration.	Oral response, discussion, and demon-stration.
UG	Exit mine	Walking tour to elevator and discuss manholes, switches, and safety guidelines for walking along the haulage.			
Day 4					
	Health – Sec. 48.5(7)	Aware of harm done by noise and silica dust, correct use of hearing protection and respirators, engineering and administrative controls for dust and noise, benefits of audiometric testing, and purpose of sampling (dust, noise, etc.). **Mine-specific:** *Will be able to demonstrate proper donning and use of the respirators and/or hearing protection provided by the mine.*	Videos, PowerPoint, discussion.	Federal stand-ards, audio-visual aids, company rules/policies.	Oral response, discussion, quizzes.

	SUBJECT	OBJECTIVES	TEACHING METHODS	COURSE MATERIAL	EVALU-ATION METHODS
	Mandatory health and safety stand-ards – Sec. 48.6(2)	Will be able to demonstrate an awareness of the most commonly violated health and safety standards and what the inspector considers when issuing a citation.	Videos, PowerPoint, discussion.	Federal stand-ards, audio-visual aids, top citation issues.	Oral response, discussion, quizzes.
	Hazard recognition – Sec. 48.5(9)	Aware of hazards and correct operating procedures. Will have participated in a job safety analysis. **Mine-specific:** *Knowledge of special hazards at the mine and operating procedures to minimize them.*	Videos, PowerPoint, discussion, mine tour.	Federal stand-ards, audio-visual aids, company rules/policies.	Oral response, discussion, quizzes.
	Electrical hazards – Sec. 48.5(10)	Aware of electrical hazards in mines, how to avoid them, and the need for lockout/tagout. **Mine-specific:** *Aware of special hazards at the mine and able to accurately explain the electrical lockout/tagout procedure in use at the mine and when/how it is applied.*	Videos, PowerPoint, discussion.	Federal stand-ards, audio-visual aids, company rules/policies.	Oral response, discussion, quizzes.
Day 5 4 hours	CPR and Automated External Defibrillator (AED) training and certifica-tion	Each attendee will participate in a 4-hour CPR and AED training session. Each will be qualified to perform in the workplace.	Video, mani-kins, AED unit, tests, and safety materials required.	American Heart Associ-ation stand-ards, video, PowerPoint program – Each will perform and test to standards for qualification.	Q&A, demonstra-tion, written and perform-ance tests.
Day 5 4 hours	First aid – Sec. 48.5(11)	Understand the importance of checking the scene to avoid personal injury, the need to get immediate help, how to perform a primary survey on the victim (check for consciousness, breathing, pulse, and severe bleeding), know about universal precautions, know how to do artificial respiration and how to control severe bleeding. **Mine-specific:** *Will know how to call emergency medical personnel and be able to direct them to the workplace.*	Videos, PowerPoint, discussion.	Federal stand-ards, audio-visual aids, company rules/policies.	Oral response, discussion, quizzes.
	Mine gases – Sec. 48.5(12)	Know about the hazardous gases typi-cally found in mine airways, when/where to expect them, the importance of ventilation, gas measurement instru-mentation calibration and reliability. **Mine-specific:** *Understand gas measurement procedures, require-ments, and actions taken when gas is encountered.*	Videos, PowerPoint, discussion.	Federal stand-ards, audio-visual aids, gas detection equipment, company rules/policies.	Oral response, discussion, quizzes.

	SUBJECT	OBJECTIVES	TEACHING METHODS	COURSE MATERIAL	EVALU-ATION METHODS
	Introduction to work environ-ment – Sec. 48.5(4)	Aware of mining methods used and associated hazards. **Mine-specific:** *Will have observed mining in progress, in particular, any unusual processes and equipment.*	Videos, PowerPoint, discussion, mine tour.	Federal stand-ards, audio-visual aids.	Oral response, discussion, quizzes.
	Information about physical and health hazards of workplace chemicals – Sec. 47(14)	Information on hazards associated with chemicals to which the miner will be exposed. **Mine-specific:** *Mine-specific chemical hazards.*	Videos, MSDSs, company program.	Videos, oral/ written ques-tions, demon-stration, or other. MSDSs.	Oral response, discussion, quizzes.
	Protective measures a miner can take against chemi-cal hazards – Sec. 47(15)	Information on protective measures the miner can take to minimize exposure to hazardous chemicals. **Mine-specific:** *Protective measures for mine-specific chemical hazards.*	Videos, MSDSs, other.	Oral/written questions, demonstra-tion, or other. MSDSs.	Oral response, discussion, quizzes.
	Contents of the mine's HazCom Program – Sec. 47(16)	Awareness of what a written HazCom Program should contain. **Mine-specific:** *Written HazCom Program.*	Videos, MSDSs, other.	Oral/written questions, demonstra-tion, or other company program.	Oral response, discussion, quizzes.
	Mandatory health and safety standards – Sec. 48.6(2)	Overview of the Act (1969 and 1977) – Most pertinent portions for new miners.	Videos, PowerPoint, discussion.	Federal stand-ards, audio-visual aids, top citations, and issues considered by MSHA.	Oral response, discussion, quizzes.
	Prevention of accidents – Sec. 48.6(8)	Aware of the major causes of serious mine accidents and correct operating procedures to prevent/minimize them. Include our SWP and Observation Program – Task training.	Videos, PowerPoint, discussion.	Federal stand-ards, audio-visual aids.	Oral response, discussion, quizzes.
	Emergency medical proce-dures – Sec. 48.6(9)	**Mine-specific:** *Will know very basic first aid and how to get immediate help in a medical emergency.* *Full-Day Training.*	Videos, PowerPoint, discussion.	Federal stand-ards, audio-visual aids, company rules/policies.	Oral response, discussion, Q&A session.

	SUBJECT	OBJECTIVES	TEACHING METHODS	COURSE MATERIAL	EVALU-ATION METHODS
	Health – Sec. 48.6(10)	Aware of harm caused by noise and silica dust, correct use of hearing protection and respirators, engineering and administrative controls for dust and noise, benefits of audiometric testing, and purpose of sampling (dust, noise, etc.). **Mine-specific:** *Will be able to demonstrate proper donning and use of respirators and/or hearing protection provided by the mine. Hearing conservation and HazCom.*	Lecture and discussion.	Federal standards, audio-visual aids, company rules/policies.	Oral response, discussion, Q&A session.
	Health and safety aspects of assigned tasks – Sec. 48.6(11)	Aware of hazards associated with common underground mine tasks. **Mine-specific:** *Know the hazards of the assigned task and procedures to minimize them.*	Lecture and discussion, demonstra-tion.	Federal standards, audio-visual aids, company and manufacturer information.	Oral response, discussion, Q&A session.
	Self-rescue and respiratory devices – Sec. 48.6(12)	Will have been instructed in the use, care, and maintenance of a self-rescuer. **Mine-specific:** *Will be fit-tested and trained in the proper use and care of any respiratory devices required at the mine, as well as self-rescuers.*	Lecture and discussion, demonstra-tion.	Federal standards, audio-visual aids, company and manufacturer information.	Oral response, discussion, Q&A session.
	Information about physical and health hazards or workplace chemicals – Sec. 47(13)	Information on hazards associated with chemicals to which the miner will be exposed. **Mine-specific:** *Mine-specific chemical hazards.*	Videos, MSDSs, company program.	Videos, oral/written questions, demon-stration, or other. MSDSs.	Oral response, discussion, quizzes.
	Protective measures a miner can take against chemi-cal hazards – Sec. 47(14)	Information on protective measures the miner can take to minimize exposure to hazardous chemicals. **Mine-specific:** *Protective measures for mine-specific chemical hazards.*	Videos, MSDSs, other.	Oral/written questions, demonstra-tion, or other. MSDSs.	Oral response, discussion, quizzes.
	Contents of the mine's HazCom Program – Sec. 47(15)	Awareness of what a written HazCom Program would contain. **Mine-specific:** *Written HazCom Program.*	Videos, MSDSs, other.	Oral/written questions, demonstra-tion, or other written program.	Oral response, discussion, quizzes.

APPENDIX C.—TASKS/DUTIES FOR TRAINING SECTION

Tasks/Duties	Expected behaviors
Entering the mine	• Outfitting of trainees, along with instructions on how to properly don their cap lights, leg bands, and other safety apparel. Cap light maintenance. • Check-in and checkout procedures, including hand scanners. • Traveling on cages, including emergencies while traveling on the cage. • Calling for a cage to exit the mine and the proper procedures. Need instructions for phone and pager usage. • How to use the mine phone at the shaft bottom.
Walking in the mine environment – safe procedures for walking, standing, or sitting in the mine	• Electrical cables and installations – Safe clearances and understanding of employees' responsibilities when working in the area of energized cables and apparatus. • Walking along and crossing rail haulage, manholes, rights of way, and general safety. • Water, slippery conditions, rough bottom, and slipping and tripping hazards. • Signs, reflectors, lights, and other indicators of travelways and dangers including stop signs, unsupported roof, and various signs and warnings. • Evaluating roof and rib conditions, including sight, sound, and vibration methods of roof testing. Scaling roof and ribs.
Shoveling in the mine environment	• Proper procedures for shoveling in the mine. Types of shovels used. Back maintenance and proper procedures. • Trainees will shovel assigned area along rib area to prepare to hang canvas and tubing. Also use of pick to prepare to set stoppings and posts. • Rock dusting
Timbering and roof control	• Trainees will evaluate roof and rib conditions, cut and set posts using an axe, shovel, measuring sticks, and saw. • Proper measurement and post installation. Axe and saw safety. • Carrying and setting cribs. Preparation, setting, wedging, and other safety considerations. • Installation of temporary jacks and permanent supports. • Safely removing posts and cribs. Area cleanup and restacking of roof support materials.
Ventilation	• Setting pogo sticks; use of wedges over straps; use of spad guns; handling, stretching, and installing canvas checks and line canvas. • Handling tubes and proper tube installation. • Tube removal and safety provisions while removing tubes. • Installation of temporary stoppings and run-through. • Removal of tubing and returning to area storage for future use.
Housekeeping	• Mantrip cleanliness. • Trash on belt. • Return tools and material. • Trash on sections. Graffiti.
Handling cables and hanging	• 300-ft sections of various cables used on section and appropriate hangers needed. Trainees will drag and hang cables according to safe job procedures. • Safe cable handling due to voltage. Never run over cables. Step on shuttle cables when crossing. Side for cables to hang, etc. High-voltage cable safety. • Use and installation of cable hangers. • Permanent electrical installations, circuit breakers, rubber mats, etc.

APPENDIX D.—TRAINING COURSE EVALUATION FORMS

Training Course Evaluation Short Form
Rev. 1.0

Course Title: _____Date:_____

Course Instructor's Name (s):_____

Use the scale on the right to indicate your opinion about each statement below.

5 = Excellent
4 = Good
3 = Fair
2 = Needs improvement
1 = Unacceptable
N/A = Not applicable

1. Relevance of the course...[....]
2. Quality of aids and materials..[....]
3. Degree of participation by trainees..[....]
4. Quality of course facilities...[....]
5. Instructor's subject knowledge...[....]
6. Overall quality of instruction...[....]
7. Instruction pace...[....]
8. Met your training needs..[....]
9. Held your interest...[....]
10. Practicality of the course..[....]
11. Amount of practice you received...[....]
12. Value of practice sessions...[....]
13. Meeting of objectives..[....]
14. Overall value of the course...[....]

Comments: _____

_____

_____

Training Course Evaluation Long Form
Rev. 1.0

Course Title: _____

Course Location: _____

Course Instructor's Name (s):_____

Your feedback is important as we seek to continuously improve the quality and efficiency of our Management Development Training Program. On a scale of 1 (Strongly Disagree) to 5 (Strongly Agree), please **circle** the number that reflects your opinion.

I. Training Course	1 Strongly Disagree	2	3	4	5 Strongly Agree
A. The course objectives were clearly stated?	1	2	3	4	5
B. The course objectives were met?	1	2	3	4	5
C. The course content was relevant to the topic?	1	2	3	4	5
D. The subject matter was well organized?	1	2	3	4	5
E. Materials used (audio visual, handouts, etc.) were beneficial in meeting the session's objectives?	1	2	3	4	5
F. The course length was appropriate?	1	2	3	4	5
G. The group activities were suitable and helpful?	1	2	3	4	5
H. Overall I feel the time we spent in training was a good investment?	1	2	3	4	5

II. The Instructor	1 Strongly Disagree	2	3	4	5 Strongly Agree
A. Effectively related subject matter to my/our learning needs?	1	2	3	4	5
B. Created a positive learning environment?	1	2	3	4	5
C. Was prepared and organized?	1	2	3	4	5
D. Covered the subject matter effectively?	1	2	3	4	5
E. Was knowledgeable of the subject matter?	1	2	3	4	5
F. Effectively kept group discussions focused on the topic?	1	2	3	4	5
G. Encouraged and managed group participation well?	1	2	3	4	5
H. Appeared interested and enthusiastic about the course?	1	2	3	4	5
I. Overall the instructor's efforts were effective?	1	2	3	4	5

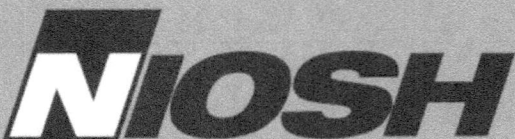

Delivering on the Nation's promise:
safety and health at work for all people
through research and prevention

To receive NIOSH documents or more information about
occupational safety and health topics, contact NIOSH at

1–800–CDC–INFO (1–800–232–4636)
TTY: 1–888–232–6348
e-mail: cdcinfo@cdc.gov

or visit the NIOSH Web site at **www.cdc.gov/niosh.**

For a monthly update on news at NIOSH, subscribe to
NIOSH *eNews* by visiting **www.cdc.gov/niosh/eNews.**

DHHS (NIOSH) Publication No. 2008–105

SAFER • HEALTHIER • PEOPLE™